About the NCCN Guidelines for Patients®

NCCN National Comprehensive Cancer Network®

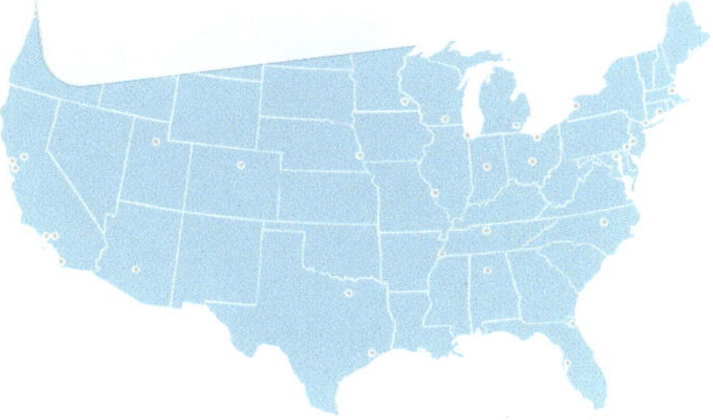

Did you know that top cancer centers across the United States work together to improve cancer care? This alliance of leading cancer centers is called the National Comprehensive Cancer Network® (NCCN®).

Cancer care is always changing. NCCN develops evidence-based cancer care recommendations used by health care providers worldwide. These frequently updated recommendations are the NCCN Clinical Practice Guidelines in Oncology (NCCN Guidelines®). The NCCN Guidelines for Patients plainly explain these expert recommendations for people with cancer and caregivers.

These NCCN Guidelines for Patients are based on the NCCN Clinical Practice Guidelines in Oncology (NCCN Guidelines®) for Chronic Lymphocytic Leukemia, Version 1.2023 – August 30, 2022.

View the NCCN Guidelines for Patients free online
NCCN.org/patientguidelines

Find an NCCN Cancer Center near you
NCCN.org/cancercenters

Connect with us

Supporters

NATIONAL COMPREHENSIVE CANCER NETWORK®
NCCN FOUNDATION
Guiding Treatment. Changing Lives.

NCCN Guidelines for Patients are supported by funding from the NCCN Foundation®

NCCN Foundation gratefully acknowledges the following corporate supporters for helping to make available these NCCN Guidelines for Patients: AbbVie, AstraZeneca, and Pharmacyclics, An AbbVie Company

NCCN independently adapts, updates and hosts the NCCN Guidelines for Patients. Our corporate supporters do not participate in the development of the NCCN Guidelines for Patients and are not responsible for the content and recommendations contained therein.

To make a gift or learn more visit online or email

NCCNFoundation.org/donate

PatientGuidelines@NCCN.org

Contents

NCCN Foundation seeks to support the millions of patients and their families affected by a cancer diagnosis by funding and distributing NCCN Guidelines for Patients. NCCN Foundation is also committed to advancing cancer treatment by funding the nation's promising doctors at the center of innovation in cancer research. For more details and the full library of patient and caregiver resources, visit NCCN.org/patients.

National Comprehensive Cancer Network (NCCN) and NCCN Foundation
3025 Chemical Road, Suite 100, Plymouth Meeting, PA 19462 USA

1
Leukemia basics

Chronic lymphocytic leukemia (CLL) is a type of blood cancer. It is unlike many other cancers because it often worsens slowly. People with CLL usually live a long time. Read this chapter to learn more about CLL. You'll find the answers to some common questions.

What is leukemia?

Leukemia is the most common type of blood cancer. It is a cancer of white blood cells or cells that become white blood cells. Also called leukocytes, white blood cells help fight germs in the body.

Leukemia cells form in bone marrow

Most bones have a soft center called marrow. Inside marrow, blood cells form from changes in a series of cells. First, blood stem cells change into either lymphoid or myeloid progenitor cells. Next, progenitor cells change into young blood cells called blasts. Healthy blasts become mature blood cells.

Types of white blood cells

White blood cells are part of myeloid and lymphoid cell lines. Basophils, neutrophils, and eosinophils are myeloid cells called granulocytes. Monocytes are another type of myeloid cell. B lymphocytes, T lymphocytes, and natural killer cells are lymphoid cells called lymphocytes.

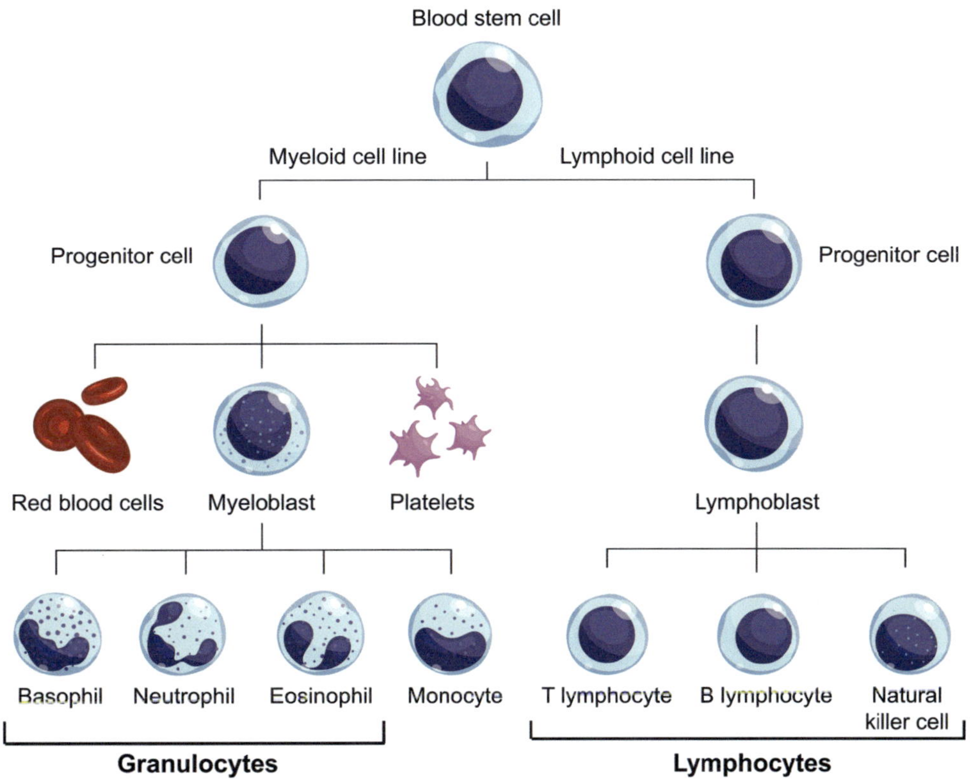

Myeloblasts are young myeloid cells that form into 2 types of white blood cells:

- Granulocytes
- Monocytes

Lymphoblasts are young lymphoid cells that form into 3 types of lymphocytes:

- B lymphocytes (also called B cells)
- T lymphocytes (T cells)
- Natural killer cells

Leukemia affects how white blood cells are made and work. It causes many abnormal white blood cells to form in bone marrow. The abnormal blood cells are called leukemia cells. Leukemia cells may fill up the bone marrow leaving little room for healthy blood cells to grow.

Leukemia cells enter the bloodstream

Normally, mature blood cells leave the bone marrow and enter the bloodstream. From the bloodstream, blood cells are released into body tissues.

Likewise, leukemia cells leave marrow and enter the bloodstream. The leukemia cells are young or partly mature blood cells. They don't work as they should.

Leukemia cells may build up in the lymph system

The bloodstream transports lymphocytes to the lymph (or lymphatic) system. The lymph system is a network of tissues that have many white blood cells and a fluid called lymph.

Lymph travels in a "superhighway" of tube-shaped vessels that are throughout the body.

Lymph system

Lymphocytes are produced in bone marrow but further develop in lymph tissue to fight disease. The tonsils, thymus, spleen, and lymph nodes are composed of lymph tissue. There are hundreds of lymph nodes in the body and many are in the neck, armpits, and groin.

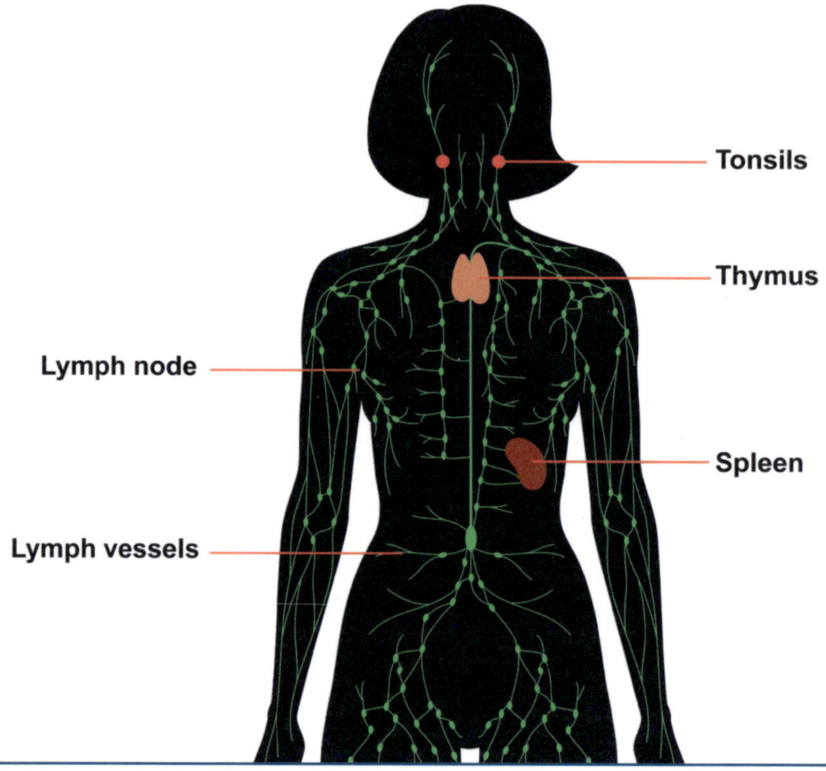

As it travels, it passes through lymph nodes (also called "glands"). Lymph nodes filter out germs and waste.

Leukemia cells may also travel into the lymph system. The leukemia cells can build up in lymph tissue causing the tissue to swell. Big lymph nodes are a common symptom of leukemia.

What is CLL?

CLL is the most common leukemia in adults. It is a cancer of B cells. The B cells look almost normal but don't function correctly. They can't fight infections well. CLL most often worsens slowly, but for some people it may worsen quickly.

How is CLL different from other leukemias?

Leukemias are divided into two groups called acute and chronic leukemias. CLL is a chronic leukemia. Chronic leukemia often worsens slowly over time. People with chronic leukemia may not have symptoms or need treatment right away. Chronic leukemia affects mature blood cells.

CLL affects lymphoid cells that make many abnormal B cells. In contrast, chronic myeloid leukemia (CML) affects the myeloid cell line. It causes many abnormal granulocytes to form.

Acute leukemia often worsens quickly and causes symptoms. Treatment is usually needed right away. Acute lymphoblastic leukemia (ALL) affects lymphoid cells that make many abnormal lymphoblasts. Acute myeloid leukemia (AML) affects myeloid cells that make many abnormal myeloblasts.

How do CLL and SLL differ?

CLL and small lymphocytic lymphoma (SLL) are the same cancer. They differ only by the location of the cancer cells.

With CLL, many leukemia cells are found in the blood and bone marrow. Leukemia cells may also be in the lymph nodes and spleen.

With SLL, there are few, if any, leukemia cells in the blood. Instead, the leukemia cells are mainly in lymph nodes and the spleen.

Treatment of CLL and SLL is very similar because the cancer cells are the same.

How is CLL found?

Most often, CLL is found because of routine blood work. A complete blood count (CBC) is a common blood test that measures the number of blood cells. A high number of lymphocytes is often the first sign of CLL.

Less often, CLL is found because of painless, swollen lymph nodes. Swollen lymph nodes often are found in multiple parts of the body. They may get smaller then get big again.

Most people don't have symptoms of CLL at diagnosis. When people do have symptoms, health care providers might not suspect cancer at first. Symptoms of CLL are caused by other health problems, too. Take fatigue, for example. It is a common symptom of CLL, but it is also caused by anemia, stress, inactivity, and some medications.

When leukemia is suspected, you'll be referred to a cancer doctor called a hematologist/oncologist. More testing is needed. Getting a diagnosis of CLL can be a shock especially if you feel healthy.

Can CLL be cured?

CLL can be treated, but it is only rarely cured. Treatment controls growth of the leukemia and reduces its signs and symptoms. For most people, though, CLL eventually worsens, and many need another round of treatment. It may take years before treatment is started or changed again.

Many people who have CLL live long lives, but life with CLL is not the same as before. You might have to live with symptoms caused by the cancer or treatment. You will need to take extra care to avoid infections.

This book explains treatment options for CLL. Treatment for CLL has greatly improved in recent years. Discuss the treatments in this book with your cancer doctor. Together, you can make a treatment plan that's best for you. Also, ask your care team about ways to improve your quality of life.

Key points

- Leukemia is a cancer of white blood cells or cells that become white blood cells. Leukemia cells are often found in the bone marrow, blood, and lymph tissue.
- CLL is a cancer of B lymphocytes. It is a chronic leukemia that often grows slowly. Treatment may not be needed right away.
- CLL and SLL are the same cancer. They differ by the location of the cancer cells. Treatment of the cancers is very similar because the cancer cells are the same.
- Tests of CLL may be done because of high lymphocyte counts, swollen nodes, or symptoms.
- Many people with CLL have normal lifespans. Living with CLL will require ongoing treatment, supportive care, and follow-up.

> "I found tremendous comfort in focusing on the things that I could control, such as taking medications as directed, taking an active role in educating myself about my disease and my treatment plan, and ensuring I asked (and received) proper answers to all my questions.

> "I found focusing and staying in touch with a small circle of close friends who really care about you helped build my mental strength. It will be easy to identify them, and the good feeling you have after a text or chat is great mental strength fuel.

2

Tests for CLL

If your health care provider suspects that you have CLL, several tests are needed. There are many types of B cell cancers, so it is important that specific tests are performed. This chapter describes the tests used to diagnose CLL and plan treatment.

Cancer tests

The only way to be sure that you have chronic lymphocytic leukemia (CLL) is to test fluid or tissue samples from your body. Most often, CLL is found (diagnosed) by testing a blood sample. The tests needed to diagnose and plan treatment are described on the next pages and are listed in **Guide 1**.

The tests for diagnosis are done at a lab. A doctor called a hematopathologist is an expert at diagnosing cancers of blood and immune cells. They spend much of their time working with samples of blood, bone marrow, and lymph tissue.

Lab results used for diagnosis are included in a pathology report. This report will be sent to your CLL doctor. Ask for a copy. It is used to plan your treatment. Your doctor will review the results with you. Take notes and ask questions.

Guide 1
Tests that everyone with CLL needs

Cancer tests	A diagnosis of CLL is made by one of these two tests: • Flow cytometry on a blood sample • IHC on biopsy samples
Genetic biomarkers	• FISH • DNA sequencing • CpG-stimulated karyotype
Health history and exam	• Medical history including B symptoms • Physical exam including spleen, liver, and areas with many lymph nodes • Performance status
Blood tests	• CBC with differential and examination of peripheral blood smear • Comprehensive metabolic panel • LDH

Diagnosis by blood test

The hematopathologist will examine a drop of your blood using a microscope. This is called a blood smear. Your oncologist may also view the blood smear. The features of the leukemia cells can be a clue as to what cancer you have.

Your blood will also be tested using a method called flow cytometry. This test shows which cells are in the blood. It can detect common patterns of proteins on the surface of cells called the immunophenotype.

Diagnosis by biopsy

A biopsy is a procedure that removes tissue samples from the body. If needed, samples of lymph nodes or bone marrow can be tested to diagnose CLL.

An excisional biopsy removes a whole lymph node, and an incisional biopsy removes part of a lymph node. Needle biopsies can be done when the other biopsies are not safe.

A method called immunohistochemistry (IHC) will be used to find the immunophenotype of the biopsied cells.

Test results needed to diagnose CLL

A diagnosis of CLL is made based on 3 test results:

- The leukemia cells have a CLL immunophenotype, which includes CD5, CD19, and CD23, some CD20, and no CD10 proteins.
- The leukemia cells are copies of the same cancer cell, which is called monoclonality.
- There are at least 5,000 monoclonal B lymphocytes in blood (5×10^9/L).

Immunophenotype

Chronic lymphocytic leukemia often has a common pattern of surface proteins on its cells. An example of these proteins is CD20 (shown). A common pattern of cell proteins is called an immunophenotype. It helps identify the correct type of cancer. For instance, CLL cells have proteins called CD200 and LEF1, but mantle cell lymphoma does not have them.

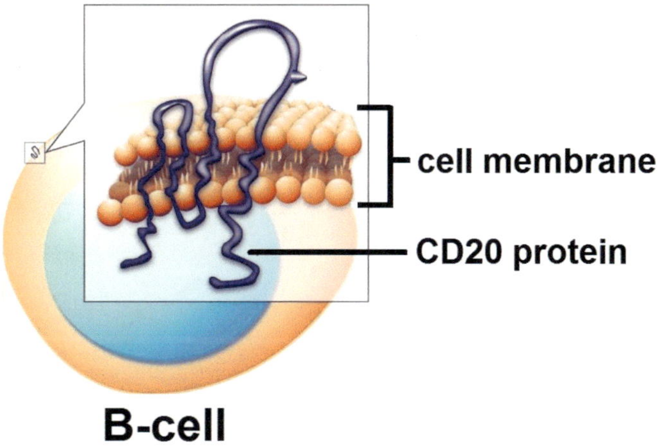

Derivative work of NIAID - Rituxima Binding to CD20 on a B Cell Surface, CC BY 2.0, https://commons.wikimedia.org/w/index.php?curid=39933221

Genetic biomarkers

Genetic information tells your cells what to do. It is located in the nucleus of a cell and stored in 46 long strands of DNA. A gene is a small segment of DNA. Strands of DNA are carried and packaged in 23 chromosomes.

Doctors look for genetic biomarkers in CLL cells. Some treatments are based on biomarkers as discussed in Chapter 5. Other biomarkers are used solely to predict the outlook (prognosis) of CLL.

Biomarkers of CLL are found with lab tests using either a blood or bone marrow sample:

- Fluorescence in situ hybridization (FISH) can show missing parts of chromosomes and extra chromosomes. In CLL, the leukemia cells may have 11q, 13q, or 17p deletions. The cells may have an extra copy of chromosome 12 also called trisomy 12.
- DNA sequencing is used to look for mutations in the *TP53* and *IGHV* genes.
- A karyotype can show defects in chromosomes. A complex karyotype is 3 or more unrelated defects in chromosomes that occur in more than one cell.

> "The key to managing fear is in making informed decisions. Stay positive, make a plan for yourself, and go forward one step at a time.

Genetic information

The nucleus is the control center or "brain" of cells. Within the nucleus is genetic information that tells the cells what to do. The information is stored in DNA, which looks like a twisted ladder. Genes are parts of DNA that contain "instructions" for the cell. At times, strands of DNA tightly coil and form into chromosomes.

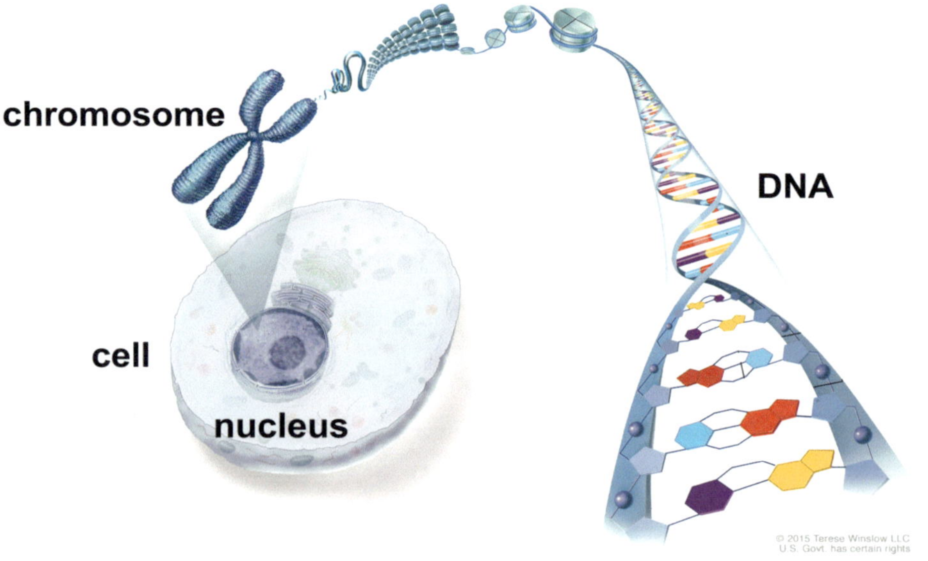

Health history

Expect your cancer care team to review your health in detail. This is known as taking a medical history. They will want to know a lot about your past and current health. You will likely be asked about:

- Illnesses (especially infections) and injuries
- Prescribed and over-the-counter medicines and supplements, surgeries, and blood transfusions
- Lifestyle choices, including your diet, how active you are, and whether you smoke or drink alcohol
- Symptoms and complications of CLL. CLL can cause “B symptoms.” B symptoms are fevers when you don't have an infection, drenching night sweats, and unexplained weight loss

Some cancers and other health conditions can run in families. Be prepared to discuss the health problems of your close blood relatives. These include brothers, sisters, parents, and grandparents. Relatives are 7 to 8 times more likely to develop CLL if there’s a family history.

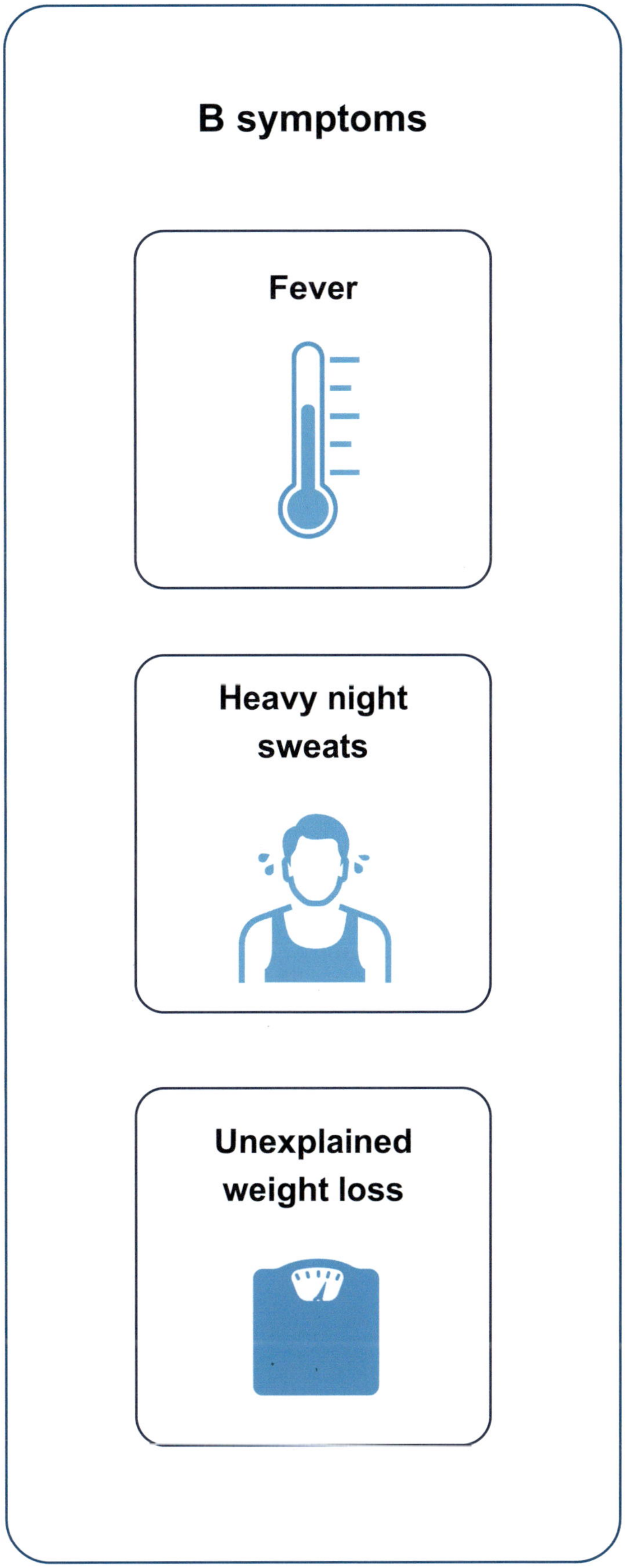

Physical exam

Your doctor will perform a thorough physical exam of your body. This exam may include:

- Checking your vital signs—blood pressure, heart rate, breathing rate, and body temperature—and assessing your overall appearance
- Feeling and listening to organs, including your spleen and liver
- Assessing your level of pain, if any, when you are touched

Checking for swelling

Leukemia cells can build up in lymph nodes, the spleen, and the liver causing them to swell. Your doctor will look at and gently press on your body to assess their size. Areas that may be touched include your neck, armpit, belly, and groin.

Checking your physical ability

Based on your history and exam, your doctor will rate your performance status. Performance status is your ability to do day-to-day activities. The Eastern Cooperative Oncology Group (ECOG) Performance Status is a common scoring system. It consists of five scores. Lower scores represent a higher ability to take care of yourself.

Blood tests

Blood tests can measure blood cells, proteins, and chemicals in the bloodstream. Samples of your blood will be removed with a needle that is inserted into a vein. This is called a blood draw. You may need to fast from food and most liquids for hours before the draw.

CBC with differential

If not done recently, a complete blood count (CBC) with differential is needed.

- A CBC measures parts of the blood including counts of white blood cells, red blood cells, and platelets.
- A differential measures the counts of the most common types of white blood cells—basophils, neutrophils, eosinophils, monocytes, and lymphocytes. It also checks if the cell counts are in balance with each other.

The white blood cell and lymphocyte counts are often high at diagnosis of CLL. Other blood counts may be low.

Comprehensive metabolic panel

A comprehensive metabolic panel is a screening test for many diseases. It often includes tests for up to 14 chemicals in the blood. Abnormal levels may mean your kidneys and liver are not working as they should.

LDH

Lactate dehydrogenase (LDH) is a protein that's in almost all cells. It can be released into your blood when a cell is damaged. A high level of LDH is an important sign of cell damage. High levels can be caused by a fast-growing cancer or other health problems.

If your LDH level is high, treatment of CLL may be needed soon.

Other blood tests

Some people with CLL may get other blood tests. Other elements in the blood that may be measured are:

- Quantitative immunoglobulins to assess your risk of infections
- Haptoglobin, reticulocytes, and Coombs tests to assess if your body is attacking your red blood cells
- Beta-2 microglobulin to assess for CLL cell growth
- Uric acid to assess the risk of tumor lysis syndrome from dying leukemia cells
- Hepatitis B antibodies and antigens since the virus could reactivate during certain cancer treatments
- Hepatitis C antibodies and antigens since the virus could affect treatment results

A complete list of tests that may be useful are listed in **Guide 2.**

Guide 2
Tests that may be useful for people with CLL

Blood tests	• Quantitative immunoglobulins • Reticulocyte count, haptoglobin, and direct antiglobulin (Coombs) test • Beta-2 microglobulin • Uric acid • Hepatitis B and hepatitis C test
Bone marrow tests	• Bone marrow biopsy and aspirate
Imaging	• Diagnostic CT of chest, abdomen, and pelvis if needed • PET/CT to guide biopsy of lymph node if Richter's transformation is suspected
Heart test	• Echocardiogram or MUGA scan if needed
Fertility and pregnancy	• Pregnancy test if needed • Fertility counseling if you're interested

Bone marrow tests

Bone marrow is the soft center in the middle of most bones. It is like a sponge holding liquid and cells. Tests on bone marrow are not often needed to diagnose CLL. However, they may be done to assess how many leukemia cells are in marrow. There are two methods of removing bone marrow.

- A bone marrow biopsy removes a core sample of the "sponge"
- A bone marrow aspiration removes liquid and cells

These procedures are often done at the same time. They're performed on the back of the hip bone. You may receive a light sedative to relax you beforehand. The samples will be sent to a hematopathologist for testing.

Imaging

Imaging takes pictures of the inside of your body. It is sometimes used to detect cancer that is deep in the body. Not all people with CLL will need imaging.

Imaging scans are done in the radiology or nuclear medicine department. A radiologist and nuclear medicine specialist are doctors who specialize in imaging. They will review your scans and send the results to your oncologist.

Diagnostic CT

Computed tomography (CT) makes a more detailed image than a plain x-ray. It takes many pictures of your body from different angles using x-rays. A computer then combines the pictures to make a 3D image.

A *diagnostic* CT shows body tissue more clearly. A higher dose of radiation is used compared to regular CT. A contrast agent (also called contrast dye) is also used to get the clearest images. Some people can't have contrast due to certain health issues. Ask your radiologist if contrast is safe for you.

Diagnostic CT of your chest, abdomen, and pelvis may be needed for two reasons. One reason is to look for big lymph nodes that may be causing symptoms. Another reason is to assess the extent of the cancer before starting a treatment called venetoclax.

PET/CT-directed needle biopsy

Sometimes CT is combined with PET (positron emission tomography). PET can detect even small amounts of cancer with a radiotracer and special camera. PET/CT is useful if your doctor thinks that CLL is turning into a fast-growing cancer called Richter's transformation If needed, PET/CT can show the best area to biopsy. The removed tissue will be tested to confirm if the leukemia has changed.

Heart test

A type of cancer drug called an anthracycline may damage your heart. It is sometimes used to treat CLL that has transformed into a faster-growing cancer. To plan treatment, your doctor may test how well your heart pumps blood.

To assess your heart, you may have an echocardiogram. An echocardiogram is an ultrasound. It uses sound waves to make pictures of the heart. The other test you may get is a multigated acquisition (MUGA) scan. A MUGA scan makes pictures using an injected radiotracer and special camera.

Fertility and pregnancy

Many people have healthy babies despite cancer and its treatment. If you wish to have a baby, there are important steps to take before treatment. Even if you are unsure, talk to your cancer care team.

Fertility counseling

Fertility is the ability to have a baby. Some cancer treatments can damage the body parts needed for fertility. Ask your cancer care team if you are at risk for impaired fertility. It can happen to people of any gender.

You may receive a referral to a fertility specialist. A fertility specialist is an expert in helping people have babies. The fertility specialist can explain how you may be able to have a baby after treatment. Collecting and freezing sperm or eggs is a common method.

More information on fertility preservation can be found at NCCN.org/PatientGuidelines and on the NCCN Patient Guides for Cancer app.

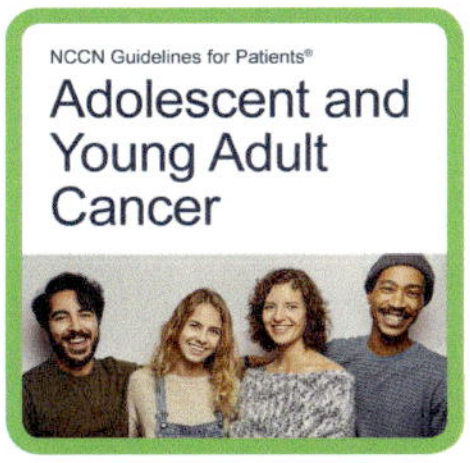

Pregnancy test

Some cancer treatments can harm an unborn baby. Your cancer care team will give you a pregnancy test before treatment if needed. Your treatment options will depend on the results.

Birth control

During treatment, don't get pregnant or get someone pregnant. Take steps to prevent pregnancy. Your cancer care team can tell you which birth control methods are best to use.

Cancer treatment can impact one's ability to have children. Before starting treatment, talk with a fertility counselor to learn what your options are for fertility preservation.

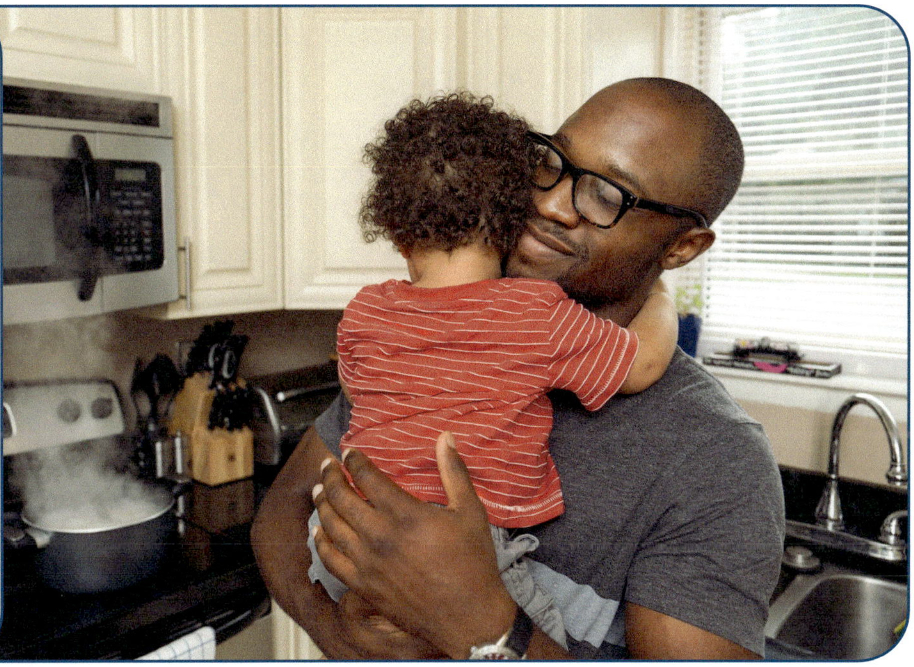

Key points

- A diagnosis of CLL is made based on tests of blood, lymph nodes, or bone marrow. Hematopathologists look for very high numbers of abnormal B cells. They also look for protein markers that are both common and uncommon to CLL cells.
- CLL doctors use genetic biomarkers to assess prognosis and plan treatment.
- Be ready to tell your cancer care team about any health problems and treatments you've had in your lifetime.
- Tell your team about any recent fevers, night sweats, and unexplained weight loss. These can be symptoms of CLL.
- Your doctor will rate your ability to do day-to-day activities in order to decide your treatment options.
- Your doctor will order blood tests and use the results to plan treatment.
- Your bone marrow may be tested to find the cause of low blood cell counts.
- Imaging allows doctors to look inside your body for cancer in tissue.
- You may have a heart test to see if you're healthy enough to have certain cancer treatments.
- Ask your cancer care team if you are at risk for impaired fertility. There are ways to have a healthy baby after cancer treatment.
- Before starting treatment, get a pregnancy test. Some cancer treatments can harm unborn babies.

share with us.

Take our survey.
And help make the
NCCN Guidelines for Patients
better for everyone!

NCCN.org/patients/comments

3
Watch and wait

CLL does not always need to be treated right away. Your care team will regularly assess the cancer and start treatment when needed. This approach is called watch and wait.

Waiting is safe

You may start treatment for CLL months or years after diagnosis. Some people never start treatment.

CLL is unlike many cancers. It often worsens very slowly. It is commonly found before it causes symptoms. Years may pass before CLL worsens to the point of needing treatment. Many people with CLL have normal lifespans.

Current research has shown that delaying treatment is safe for many people. Ongoing research is testing whether to delay or start newer treatments of CLL. Reasons to delay treatment include:

- Early treatment of CLL does not lengthen life
- Treatment may cause health problems called side effects
- There may be better treatments in the future

Wellness while you wait

Watch and wait is a period of testing for changes in cancer status. It is also called observation, active surveillance, and watchful waiting. During watch and wait, your cancer care team will monitor your symptoms and blood counts. Watch and wait can go on for years.

During watch and wait, you can take care of your health in several ways. First, go to your health appointments. Do not skip or delay them. Second, find support. Watch and wait can cause worry or anxiety. Support groups or professional support may be helpful. Third, live a healthy lifestyle to improve your overall health.

NCCN has resources to help you during watch and wait. NCCN has a two-part book series on survivorship care. One survivorship book gives recommendations on healthy living. The other book focuses on cancer symptoms, such as fatigue and poor sleep.

NCCN also has a book on distress. Everyone with cancer has some distress at some point in time. Distress is normal. The NCCN book explains when you're likely to be distressed and how to get relief.

The NCCN books on survivorship care and distress can be found at NCCN.org/PatientGuidelines and on the NCCN Patient Guides for Cancer app.

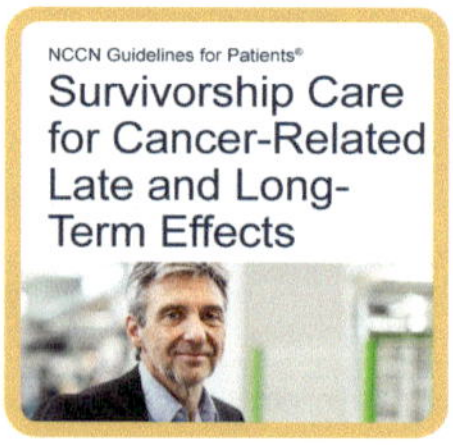

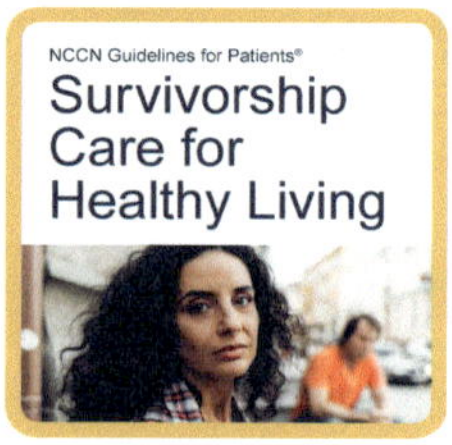

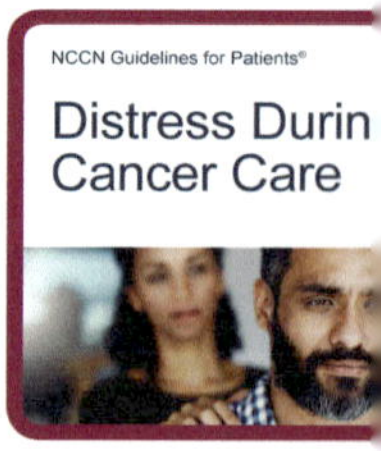

When to start treatment

It's important to talk with your cancer doctor about starting treatment. Share your wishes and concerns. Your doctor will track the cancer stage, signs, and symptoms. Together, you can decide when it's time to start treatment.

Rai stages

A cancer stage is a rating by your cancer doctor that suggests the outcome of the cancer. The Rai staging system is commonly used for CLL. It consists of 5 cancer stages ranging from stage 0 to stage 4. Often, the stages are written with Roman numerals—stages 0, I, II, III, and IV.

The Rai staging system is based on how lymphocytes are affecting the body. In all stages, there are many abnormal lymphocytes in the body. In stage 0, the lymphocytes are not having a major effect on lymphoid tissue, the liver, or bone marrow. In stages 1 and 2, the lymphocytes are causing swelling of the lymph nodes, spleen, or liver. In stages 3 or 4, the lymphocytes in bone marrow are causing a drop in the number of red blood cells or platelets. The criteria for each stage are listed in **Guide 3.**

The 5 stages can be condensed into three risk groups:

- Stage 0 has a **low risk** of getting worse.
- Stages 1 and 2 have an **intermediate risk** of getting worse.
- Stages 3 and 4 have a **high risk** of getting worse.

Guide 3
Criteria for Rai stages of CLL

	Rai 0	Rai 1	Rai 2	Rai 3	Rai 4
Many lymphocytes (lymphocytosis)	●	●	●	●	●
Enlarged lymph nodes (lymphadenopathy)		●	○	○	○
Enlarged spleen, liver, or both (organomegaly)			●	○	○
Low numbers of red blood cells (anemia)				●	○
Low numbers of platelets (thrombocytopenia)					●

● required criterion ○ may occur

Reasons to treat

In general, treatment is started when the effects of cancer become worse than the risks of its treatment. At this point, treatment may make you feel better. A high white blood cell count by itself is not a reason to treat CLL. Reasons to start treatment are listed by Rai stage in **Guide 4.**

Rai stage 0, stage 1, and stage 2 are early stages of CLL. Early-stage CLL often does not need to be treated right away. Treatment is started when there are major signs or symptoms that the cancer is getting worse. Another reason to start treatment is enrollment in an open clinical trial. A clinical trial is a type of health research. There may be a trial of new ways to treat CLL.

Rai stage 3 and stage 4 are advanced stages of CLL. Treatment is started when one or more blood cell counts are low and keep dropping. You may be able to delay treatment if your counts aren't too low and don't drop more.

Guide 4
Reasons to start treatment

Rai stage 0 **Rai stage 1** **Rai stage 2**	You can enroll in a clinical trial
	You have major symptoms of CLL • Severe fatigue • Drenching night sweats • Unintended loss of at least 10 percent of your body weight within 6 months • Fever without an infection
	CLL is causing one or more of your organs to stop working properly
	The size of your spleen or lymph nodes is growing quickly or causing discomfort
	CLL is causing the number of red blood cells to decrease
	CLL is causing the number of platelets to decrease
	Your body is killing your blood cells (autoimmune cytopenia) and treatment with steroids is not working
Rai stage 3 **Rai stage 4**	The number of blood cells is low (cytopenia) and getting lower

Key points

- Early treatment of CLL does not lengthen life. Clinical trials are testing if starting new treatments early will improve results.
- Your doctors will regularly check the status of CLL during watch and wait.
- You can take care of your health by going to appointments, finding support, and living healthfully.
- Treatment is started based on your wishes and the stage, signs, and symptoms of CLL.

"

Meeting with and learning from other CLL patients is one of the best sources of emotional and educational support that I have seen. In a CLL support group, we can share our feelings, experiences, and encouragement with the only ones who are able to see CLL from the inside out - the patients!

4

Advances in treatment

There have been several breakthroughs in the treatment of CLL. Newer treatments are better at controlling the cancer and improving quality of life. Despite improved treatment, a cure is still needed. Better treatments are made possible with clinical trials.

Going beyond chemotherapy

Chemotherapy is a term for drugs that kill rapidly dividing cells. In general, cancer cells rapidly divide but so do some healthy cells. Chemotherapy alone was once the standard treatment of CLL. Sometimes, it didn't have great results. It also can be harsh on the body because it is not as targeted as other treatments and can kill a broad range of healthy cells.

Treatment for CLL has greatly improved in recent years. Newer treatments target how leukemia cells live, survive, and die. These treatments also affect healthy cells less so than chemotherapy. This section briefly describes some of the advances in treatment.

Antibody therapy

Antibodies are proteins made by the body but can also be made in a lab to treat cancer. Antibody therapy marks leukemia cells so that the immune system can find and destroy them. It is a type of immunotherapy. When used with chemotherapy, the treatment is called chemoimmunotherapy.

- Obinutuzumab (Gazyva) and rituximab (Rituxan) bind to CD20 proteins on B cells
- Alemtuzumab (Campath) binds to CD52 proteins on T cells and B cells

BCR pathway blockers

The B cell receptor (BCR) is a protein on the surface of B cells. It triggers a chemical pathway in B cells that tells the cells to stay alive and make new cells. Cancer drugs that block proteins in the BCR pathway cause the cells to die.

- Acalabrutinib (Calquence), ibrutinib (Imbruvica), and zanubrutinib (Brukinsa) block Bruton's tyrosine kinase (BTK) and are called BTK inhibitors
- Idelalisib (Zydelig) and duvelisib (Copiktra) are PI3K inhibitors

BCL-2 pathway blockers

BCL-2 is a protein inside of B cells that helps prevent cell death. In CLL, BCL-2 may build up and stop the cancer cells from dying. BCL-2 inhibitors allow the leukemia cells to self-destruct. The BCL-2 inhibitor used to treat CLL is:

- Venetoclax (Venclexta)

How to improve treatment

Despite advances in treatment, more research is needed because current treatments rarely cure CLL. Without a cure, many people live with side effects from long-term treatment. Other people stop treatment then restart when CLL worsens. People with CLL are at risk of life-threatening infections.

Clinical trials

A clinical trial is a type of medical research study. After being developed and tested in a laboratory, potential new ways of fighting cancer need to be studied in people. If found to be safe and effective in a clinical trial, a drug, device, or treatment approach may be approved by the U.S. Food and Drug Administration (FDA).

Everyone with cancer should carefully consider all of the treatment options available for their cancer type, including standard treatments and clinical trials. Talk to your doctor about whether a clinical trial may make sense for you.

Phases

Most cancer clinical trials focus on treatment. Treatment trials are done in phases.

- **Phase I trials** study the dose, safety, and side effects of an investigational drug or treatment approach. They also look for early signs that the drug or approach is helpful.
- **Phase II trials** study how well the drug or approach works against a specific type of cancer.
- **Phase III trials** test the drug or approach against a standard treatment. If the

Finding a clinical trial

In the United States

NCCN Cancer Centers
NCCN.org/cancercenters

The National Cancer Institute (NCI)
cancer.gov/about-cancer/treatment/clinical-trials/search

Worldwide

The U.S. National Library of Medicine (NLM)
clinicaltrials.gov/

Need help finding a clinical trial?

NCI's Cancer Information Service (CIS)
1.800.4.CANCER (1.800.422.6237)
cancer.gov/contact

results are good, it may be approved by the FDA.

- **Phase IV trials** study the long-term safety and benefit of an FDA-approved treatment.

ho can enroll?

very clinical trial has rules for joining, called igibility criteria. The rules may be about age, ncer type and stage, treatment history, or neral health. These requirements ensure at participants are alike in specific ways d that the trial is as safe as possible for the rticipants.

formed consent

linical trials are managed by a group of perts called a research team. The research am will review the study with you in detail, cluding its purpose and the risks and nefits of joining. All of this information is also ovided in an informed consent form. Read e form carefully and ask questions before gning it. Take time to discuss it with family, ends, or others you trust. Keep in mind that u can leave and seek treatment outside of e clinical trial at any time.

tart the conversation

on't wait for your doctor to bring up clinical als. Start the conversation and learn about of your treatment options. If you find a study at you may be eligible for, ask your treatment am if you meet the requirements. If you have ready started standard treatment, you may t be eligible for certain clinical trials. Try t to be discouraged if you cannot join. New nical trials are always becoming available.

Frequently asked questions

There are many myths and misconceptions surrounding clinical trials. The possible benefits and risks are not well understood by many with cancer.

Will I get a placebo?
Placebos (inactive versions of real medicines) are almost never used alone in cancer clinical trials. It is common to receive either a placebo with a standard treatment or a new drug with a standard treatment. You will be informed, verbally and in writing, if a placebo is part of a clinical trial before you enroll.

Are clinical trials free?
There is no fee to enroll in a clinical trial. The study sponsor pays for research-related costs, including the study drug. You may, however, have costs indirectly related to the trial, such as the cost of transportation or child care due to extra appointments. During the trial, you will continue to receive standard cancer care. This care is billed to—and often covered by—insurance. You are responsible for copays and any costs for this care that are not covered by your insurance.

Key points

- Several advances in CLL treatment have been made. Newer treatments include immunotherapy and BTK, PI3K, and BCL-2 inhibitors.
- Despite advances in treatment, a cure for CLL is still needed.
- Clinical trials test potential new ways of fighting cancer in people.
- Ask your treatment team about the option of a clinical trial.

5
Treatment and support

Not everyone with CLL receives the same treatment. Discuss the options in this chapter with your doctor. Your doctor will tailor treatment to you and the cancer you have.

Biomarker-based treatment

CLL differs between people. Differences in how CLL behaves are caused by abnormal changes in cancer cells called biomarkers. Because biomarkers differ between people, a treatment that helps one person might not help you. That's why it's important to have biomarker testing and get a treatment plan specific to you.

Some biomarkers may change during watch and wait. Biomarkers may also change after treatment starts. Before each line of treatment, your doctor should test the cancer cells again for biomarkers. There are 4 important lab tests:

- Fluorescence in situ hybridization (FISH) for 17p deletion
- DNA sequencing for *TP53* mutation
- DNA sequencing for *IGHV* mutation if not done before
- CpG-stimulated karyotype for complex genetic changes

17p deletion

One biomarker that differs between people with CLL is called 17p deletion. A 17p deletion is a missing part of chromosome 17. It is sometimes written as del(17p). When 17p is deleted, a gene called *TP53* is deleted, too.

The *TP53* gene contains instructions for building a protein called p53. The p53 protein is needed to repair damaged DNA and start the process for cells beyond repair to die. p53 is absent in CLL cells if there is a 17p deletion. When absent, chemotherapy will likely not be an effective treatment.

TP53 mutation

In CLL cells that have 17p, the *TP53* gene may be mutated. A mutated *TP53* gene causes the p53 protein to be abnormal and not work as it should. When mutated, chemotherapy will likely not be an effective treatment.

IGHV mutation

Mutations in leukemia cells are almost always a bad thing. One exception is mutated *IGHV* region genes that cause mutated IGHV receptors. These mutations mean the leukemia cells may have formed from more mature B cells. When B cells are more mature, CLL worsens more slowly and responds better to chemotherapy. If not done before, testing for *IGHV* mutation status is needed before treatment.

Complex karyotype

A complex karyotype is 3 or more unrelated defects in chromosomes that occur in more than one cell. A complex karyotype suggests worse outcomes, but more research is needed. Prognosis may depend on the type of defect, number of defects, and combination of defects in the cells. In fact, some complex karyotypes may suggest a good outcome. But, in general, a complex karyotype may limit how well Bruton's tyrosine kinase (BTK) inhibitors work.

Options for first-line therapy

The first treatment given is referred to as first-line therapy. Before starting treatment, you may undergo imaging. Imaging is done to see if lymph nodes, the spleen, and the liver are enlarged. Doctors use imaging to make decisions about cancer treatment and the outlook.

Planning treatment

There are multiple good treatment options for CLL. Your doctor will plan treatment for you based on:

- Your age, overall health, and medications
- Biomarkers
- Length of remission that is typically achieved by treatments
- Your wishes for time-limited treatment and at-home treatment

A key factor for deciding treatment options is whether there is a 17p deletion or *TP53* mutation. These biomarkers are uncommon in people with CLL who have not had treatment. The recommendations of NCCN experts for first-line therapy based on biomarkers and other factors are discussed next.

Clinical trials

Clinical trials are a type of research. Within clinical trials, new ways of treating cancer are tested. Treatment of CLL has greatly improved because of clinical trials.

More clinical trials are needed to find better ways to treat CLL. The order in which different treatments are being used is changing. Research on combinations of treatment is ongoing.

NCCN experts recommend clinical trials, especially if the CLL cells have 17p deletion or a *TP53* mutation. Even with newer treatments, outcomes for CLL with either marker are worse than other CLL types. Clinical trials are key to finding better treatments.

Preferred regimens

A regimen consists of one or more cancer drugs. Preferred regimens work well and are the safest. The preferred regimens are almost the same for CLL with or without a 17p deletion or *TP53* mutation. **See Guide 5 and Guide 6** for a list of regimens for first-line therapy.

BTK inhibitors

BTK inhibitors are central to the treatment of CLL. They block signals from the B cell receptor (BCR). They are pills and can be taken at home. They are taken for as long as they are working.

Acalabrutinib is a newer BTK inhibitor. It may be combined with obinutuzumab, which is an immunotherapy. Obinutuzumab is slowly injected into a vein (called an infusion) at a health care center.

Zanubrutinib is the newest BTK inhibitor. It is used by itself to treat CLL. It may be an option when other BTK inhibitors cause troubling side effects.

Venetoclax regimens

Venetoclax is a newer first-line therapy. It is a BCL-2 inhibitor and may be combined with obinutuzumab. Venetoclax is a pill and can be taken at home.

Some people with CLL may prefer venetoclax over BTK inhibitors. Venetoclax is taken for 1 year and reduces CLL to very low levels.

aking venetoclax for a fixed time may prevent LL from becoming resistant to it.

)ther recommended regimens

here are important differences in other egimens based on biomarkers but also ommonly used regimens. For example, rutinib may be used whether CLL has a 17p eletion or *TP53* mutation or not. It was the first BTK inhibitor used to treat CLL. It often has very good results but can cause serious side effects including heart disease. Important regimen differences between biomarker groups are discussed next.

CLL *without* 17p deletion and *TP53* mutation

For CLL without 17p deletion and *TP53* mutation, your age and overall health may

Guide 5
First-line regimens for CLL *without* 17p deletion and TP53 mutation

Preferred regimens	• Acalabrutinib with or without obinutuzumab • Venetoclax and obinutuzumab • Zanubrutinib
Other recommended regimens	• Ibrutinib • Bendamustine and either rituximab or obinutuzumab • Chlorambucil and obinutuzumab • Obinutuzumab
Sometimes useful regimens	Fludarabine, cyclophosphamide, and rituximab (FCR) may be used to treat CLL with *IGHV* mutations in peope who are under 65 years of age and fairly healthy

Guide 6
First-line regimens for CLL *with* 17p deletion and TP53 mutation

Preferred regimens	• Acalabrutinib with or without obinutuzumab • Venetoclax with or without obinutuzumab • Zanubrutinib
Other recommended regimens	• Alemtuzumab with or without rituximab • High-dose methylprednisolone (HDMP) and rituximab • Ibrutinib • Obinutuzumab

affect which regimens are options for you. Take chemoimmunotherapy, for instance. You must be healthy enough to take this treatment since it can cause severe side effects. An alkylating agent—bendamustine or chlorambucil—with a CD20 antibody is commonly used. Fludarabine, cyclophosphamide, and rituximab (FCR) works well in a subset of people.

There are more options that need further research. Research on ibrutinib with obinutuzumab, rituximab, or venetoclax is ongoing.

CLL *with* 17p deletion and *TP53* mutation
For CLL with 17p deletion or *TP53* mutation, chemotherapy does not work well. Treatment with BTK inhibitors or CD20 or CD52 antibodies has better results. Ibrutinib with venetoclax may be an option, but more research is needed.

Supportive care

Supportive care aims to improve your quality of life. It is sometimes called palliative care. It is a key part of cancer care for everyone, not just people at the end of life. Talk with your treatment team to get the best supportive care for you.

Supportive care can address many needs. One common part of supportive care is treating health problems caused by cancer or cancer treatment, which are often simply called "side effects." Some of these health problems are listed in **Guide 7** and are discussed next.

Preventing infections

You are more likely to get infections due to CLL or its treatment. Here are some recommendations in regard to infections:

- You can protect yourself by being up-to-date on your vaccines. Recommended vaccines are listed in Guide 7. NCCN offers more information on COVID-19 at NCCN.org/covid-19.
- For frequent infections in your ear, sinuses, or lungs, immunoglobulin infusions may help prevent new infections.
- You can take medicines that help to prevent herpes and pneumocystis jiroveci pneumonia infections. These infections are more likely when treated with purine analog- or bendamustine-based chemoimmunotherapy or alemtuzumab.

Be aware of possible side effects. Your cancer care team can inform you of what to expect. Tell them right away about any new or worse symptoms.

Guide 7
Supportive care

Flu	• Influenza vaccine every year but not the live, attenuated type
Pneumococcal infection	• Pneumococcal polysaccharide vaccine (PPSV23) every 5 years or when prescribed by your provider • If you haven't yet received PPSV23, you may get the pneumococcal conjugate vaccine (PCV20) first
Shingles	• Recombinant, adjuvanted zoster vaccine before starting treatment or if on a BTK inhibitor
COVID-19	• COVID-19 vaccines to prevent serious illness • Wear a mask, keep a distance from others, and wash your hands to prevent getting infected by the COVID-19 virus • Your doctor may prescribe tixagevimab and cilgavimab (Evusheld) to prevent severe COVID-19
Frequent, severe infections of ears, sinuses, or lungs	• Antimicrobials as needed (for example, antibiotics) • If IgG is less than 500 mg/dL, infusions of immunoglobulin into a vein or skin every month
Herpes	• Prevent with a drug like acyclovir
Pneumocystis jiroveci pneumonia	• Prevent with drugs like sulfamethoxazole and trimethoprim
Hepatitis B reactivation	• Prevent or treat with entecavir or other antivirals
Cytomegalovirus reactivation	• Take ganciclovir if virus is present or rising
Hepatitis C	• Treat with direct-acting antiviral agents
Cancer	• Get screened for new cancers as needed
Autoimmune cytopenia	• Treat with corticosteroids, rituximab, IVIG, cyclosporin A, splenectomy, eltrombopag, romiplostim, Bruton's tyrosine kinase (BTK) inhibitors
Tumor lysis syndrome	• Prevent with hydration, managing hyperuricemia, and taking allopurinol, febuxostat, or rasburicase
Blood clot	• Prevent with aspirin if taking lenalidomide and not on an anticoagulant
Tumor flare reaction	• Prevent with steroids if lymph nodes are enlarged and treat with steroids and antihistamines
Blood transfusion needed	• Transfusion should be done according to hospital standards; all blood products should be radiated

Hepatitis and cytomegalovirus

If you've had hepatitis B or cytomegalovirus, these viruses may be reactivated during cancer treatment. Hepatitis B may be reactivated when taking CD20 antibodies or chemotherapy. Cytomegalovirus may be reactivated when taking PI3K inhibitors and alemtuzumab. Reactivation may be prevented with antiviral medications.

There is a link between hepatitis C and B-cell non-Hodgkin lymphomas. Direct-acting antiviral agents safely treat hepatitis C and may reduce lymphoma cells.

Cancer

People with CLL are at higher risk for other cancers, so it is important to get regular cancer screening. There are screening programs for prostate, breast, cervical, lung, and colorectal cancers. People with CLL are also at risk for non-melanoma skin cancers. See a dermatologist once a year and protect your skin from the sun.

Autoimmune cytopenia

Autoimmune cytopenia is a condition in which your immune system attacks your blood cells. There are several types of autoimmune cytopenias. Autoimmune hemolytic anemia, immune-mediated thrombocytopenia, and pure red blood cell aplasia are the most common among people with CLL. Several treatment options are listed in Guide 7.

Tumor lysis syndrome

Some treatments for CLL kill many cells quickly, such as:

- Chemoimmunotherapy
- Venetoclax
- Lenalidomide
- Obinutuzumab

Tumor lysis syndrome occurs when the waste released by dead cells is not quickly cleared out of the body. This may result in kidney damage and severe blood electrolyte disturbances. It can be life threatening.

Tumor lysis syndrome may be prevented with hydration. Drink lots of water. You may also get fluid infused into your bloodstream. Medicines that lower uric acid can help, too. See Guide 7. Some people are admitted to the hospital before starting treatment.

Blood clots and tumor flare

Lenalidomide may cause blood clots and tumor flare. A blood clot is a gel-like clump of blood that may block blood vessels. Tumor flare is a fast, short-lived increase in cancer growth. Symptoms of tumor flare include enlarged lymph nodes or spleen, low fever, and rash. Medicines that prevent and treat blood clots and tumor flare are listed in Guide 7.

Blood transfusion

Some people being treated for CLL will need a blood transfusion. The transfusion should be done according to hospital standards. All blood should be treated with radiation before the transfusion. This will prevent the rare event of transfused blood attacking your body.

Checking treatment results

You will need to have tests to assess treatment results. These tests include an updated medical history and physical exam, blood work, and sometimes imaging. There are four types of treatment results based on these tests:

- **Complete remission** is the best result. With a complete remission, enlarged organs and lymph nodes are back to normal size. You have no leukemia symptoms like fever. Blood counts are within normal range. No leukemia cells are detected in the bone marrow with common tests.
- **Partial remission** is a good result. Enlarged organs and nodes have shrunk to less than half their size. Blood counts are returning to normal.
- **Stable disease** is less than a partial remission. The cancer is not getting worse.
- **Progressive disease** is a worsening of the cancer.

Minimal residual disease

During or after treatment, your doctor may also look for tiny amounts of leukemia cells in blood called minimal residual disease (MRD). Sometimes, there are so few leukemia cells that a special test is needed to detect them. The three tests used to detect MRD include:

- Allele-specific oligonucleotide polymerase chain reaction (ASO-PCR)
- Six-color flow cytometry (MRD flow)
- Next-generation DNA sequencing (NGS)-based assays

NGS-based assays are especially good at finding leukemia cells. They can find 1 leukemia cell within 1 million cells.

A finding of *undetectable* MRD means the special test detected no leukemia cells. There may be no leukemia cells or too few to be found. Despite these great results, CLL may not be cured.

Undetectable MRD may predict the results of treatment better than a complete response. Research supports the use of MRD testing to assess treatment results.

CLL in remission

When remission is achieved, your doctor will monitor the status of CLL. You will have regular visits with your treatment team. CLL tends to worsen over time, but it may take years before the next treatment is needed. The return of leukemia is called a relapse.

After achieving remission with BCR inhibitors, keep taking the treatment. Over time, the leukemia cells may mutate and stop treatment from working. A different treatment will be started quickly if relapse occurs.

Chemoimmunotherapy and venetoclax are received for a limited time. Treatment is stopped once the cancer is in remission. During remission, your care will consist of "watch and wait." Also called observation or watchful waiting, it is a period of testing to assess for changes in cancer status. If the cancer returns, treatment is started when there are signs that it is needed.

Options after first-line therapy

It is very common for CLL to be treated with multiple lines of therapy. Second-line therapy is the second drug regimen to be tried. Third-line therapy is received after first- and second-line therapies have been tried.

There are two reasons that another line of therapy is needed. The first reason is that a therapy didn't work. In this case, the cancer is described as "refractory," and a different regimen is received. The second reason for another line of therapy is a cancer relapse. For a relapse, your doctor may give the same or a different treatment than was given before.

You may have multiple treatment options among the ones listed in this section. Your doctor will plan the next line of therapy based on many factors:

- Your overall health, medications, and preferences
- Previously known biomarkers
- New biomarkers, such as *BTK* and *PLCG2* mutations, which may make BTK inhibitors not work
- Previous types of treatment and their side effects
- Results of prior therapy and how long the results lasted

Clinical trial

A clinical trial may be an option. The best order of current treatments is being studied. There may be a clinical trial of a new cancer drug. Ask your cancer care team if there is a clinical trial that is a good fit for you.

Recommended regimens

Recommended regimens after first-line therapy are based on whether CLL has a 17p deletion or *TP53* mutation.

CLL *without* 17p deletion and *TP53* mutation

When starting a new line of therapy, treatment is often switched from one type of drug to a different type. Switching from a BTK inhibitor to venetoclax or from venetoclax to a BTK inhibitor is common. If you had first-line chemoimmunotherapy or immunotherapy, treatment may be switched to a BTK inhibitor or venetoclax. **See Guide 8** for preferred regimens and other options.

Sometimes, switching to a different type of cancer drug is not needed. If a first-line BTK inhibitor caused severe side effects, you may be able to try a different BTK inhibitor. If remission was achieved with first-line venetoclax and obinutuzumab, you may be able to take this regimen again for second-line therapy.

BTK inhibitors and venetoclax regimens are often used early in treatment. After they have been used, the next options include PI3K inhibitors, chemoimmunotherapy, or immunotherapy. You must be healthy enough to take chemoimmunotherapy since it may cause serious side effects. More research on HDMP plus a CD20 antibody is needed. **See Guide 9** for a list of recommended regimens.

CLL *with* 17p deletion and *TP53* mutation

Preferred regimens include the BTK inhibitors acalabrutinib and zanubrutinib. Ibrutinib is also an option but can cause serious side effects. If a BTK inhibitor stopped working because of a mutation, a different one may not work either.

Guide 8
Second- and third-line regimens for CLL *without* 17p deletion and *TP53* mutation

When your prior treatment consisted of a BTK inhibitor, your options may be:

- Venetoclax and rituximab (preferred) or venetoclax if not received before
- For some people, one of these BTK inhibitors—if not received before—may be an option: acalabrutinib (preferred), zanubrutinib (preferred), or ibrutinib

When your prior treatment consisted of venetoclax, your options may be:

- Repeating first-line venetoclax with obinutuzumab for second-line therapy if the cancer had been in remission
- Acalabrutinib (preferred), zanubrutinib (preferred), or ibrutinib

When your prior treatment consisted of chemoimmunotherapy or immunotherapy, your options may be:

- Venetoclax and rituximab (preferred) or venetoclax
- Acalabrutinib (preferred), zanubrutinib (preferred), or ibrutinib

Guide 9
Regimens after taking BTK inhibitors and venetoclax for CLL *without* 17p deletion and *TP53* mutation

- Duvelisib
- Idelalisib with or without rituximab
- Bendamustine and rituximab
- Fludarabine, cyclophosphamide, and rituximab (FCR)
- Lenalidomide with or without rituximab
- Obinutuzumab

Venetoclax regimens are also a preferred treatment. They may be an option if BTK inhibitors stopped working because the CLL cells have mutated.

There is a wide range of other options. Your doctor may recommend taking a CD20 or CD52 antibody. PI3K inhibitors are also used for second- and third-line regimens. The immunomodulatory agent, lenalidomide, may also be an option for you. **See Guide 10** for a complete list of recommended regimens.

Stem cell transplant

A hematopoietic stem cell is a cell in the bone marrow that develops into every type of blood cell. An allogeneic hematopoietic stem cell transplant forms new, healthy bone marrow that makes healthy blood cells. An allogeneic transplant uses healthy stem cells from a donor.

Your doctor may discuss allogeneic stem cell transplant with you. It may be an option if other treatments for CLL stop working well. You must not have major health problems other than the cancer.

There are several steps to receiving an allogeneic transplant. You may stay on cytoreductive treatment to reduce spleen size and improve symptoms until you get a transplant.

Step 1 – Your blood will be tested for cell proteins called human leukocyte antigens (HLAs). HLAs mark your cells so your body knows which cells are yours. A donor's HLA type must be a near-perfect match to yours for a transplant to work. Otherwise, your body will reject the donor stem cells or the donor cells will attack your body. Even with a near-perfect match, donor cells may attack your body. This is called graft-versus-host disease (GVHD).

Step 2 – You'll receive treatment called *conditioning* to kill your bone marrow cells. Conditioning creates room for the healthy stem cells. It also weakens the immune system so your body does not kill the donor cells. Conditioning usually involves chemotherapy.

Guide 10
Second- and third-line regimens for CLL *with* 17p deletion and TP53 mutation

Preferred regimens	• Acalabrutinib • Venetoclax with rituximab • Venetoclax • Zanubrutinib
Other regimens	• Ibrutinib • Alemtuzumab with or without rituximab • Duvelisib • High-dose methylprednisolone (HDMP) and rituximab • Idelalisib with or without rituximab • Lenalidomide with or without rituximab

Radiation therapy is sometimes used by itself or with chemotherapy.

Step 3 – Next, you'll receive the donor cells through a transfusion. A transfusion is a slow injection of blood products into a vein. The donor cells will travel to your bone marrow, rest there, and grow. They will also attack cancer cells that weren't killed by prior treatment. New, healthy blood cells will form over the next 2 to 4 weeks. This is called engraftment.

Step 4 – You'll have to be extra careful to avoid germs for the first few weeks after the transplant. That's because your infection-fighting immune system will be almost gone. You may stay in a very clean room at the hospital or be given antibiotics to prevent or treat infection. You may receive medicine called immunosuppressants to prevent GVHD. While waiting for the cells to engraft, you will likely feel tired and weak.

More information on GVHD can be found at NCCN.org/PatientGuidelines and on the NCCN Patient Guides for Cancer app.

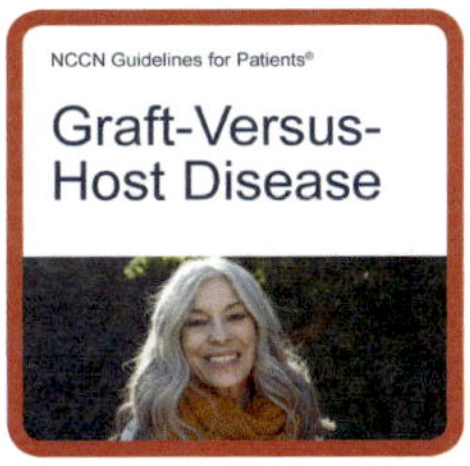

Get to know your care team and let them get to know you.

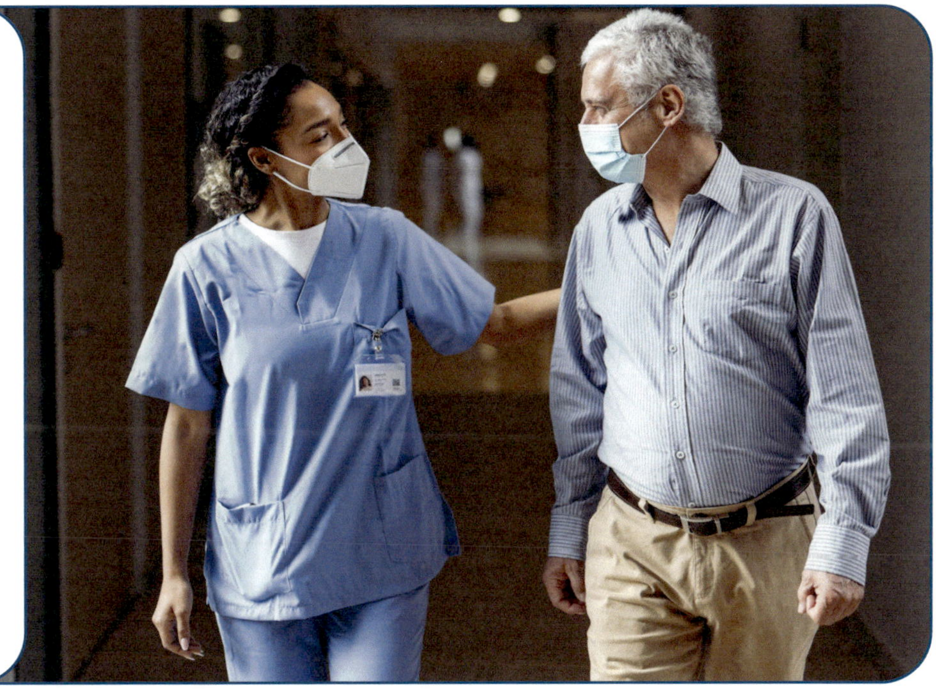

Richter's transformation

A few people with CLL develop a faster-growing lymphoma. This change is called Richter's transformation or Richter's syndrome. The new lymphoma can evolve from mutations within CLL cells or from another B cell. Richter's transformation can occur before or after treatment of CLL.

Testing is needed to confirm Richter's transformation. A biopsy of lymph nodes will be done. The removed cells will be assessed for marker proteins on their surface. Blood tests and imaging will be done, too.

CLL most often transforms into diffuse large B-cell lymphoma (DLBCL). Less often, it changes into Hodgkin lymphoma.

DLBCL

Treatment options depend on if the DLBCL cells evolved from CLL cells. If DLBCL did not evolve from CLL cells, the lymphoma is treated as DLBCL. Treatment of DLBCL can be found at NCCN.org/PatientGuidelines and on the NCCN Patient Guides for Cancer app.

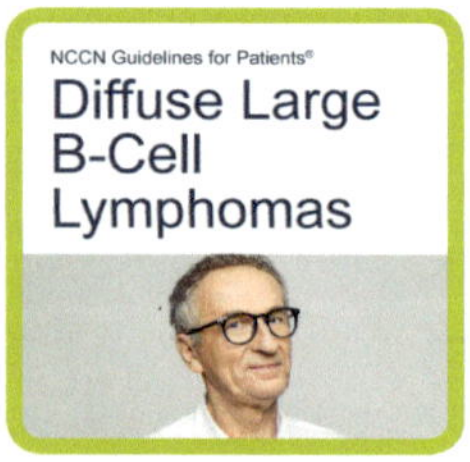

For DLBCL that evolved from CLL cells, a clinical trial is preferred. Another option is rituximab-based chemoimmunotherapy. If chemoimmunotherapy works, you may receive an allogeneic transplant if you are healthy enough. Otherwise, the next options include treatment of DLBCL.

Hodgkin lymphoma

A clinical trial is a preferred treatment option. Another option is treatment used for Hodgkin lymphoma. Treatment of Hodgkin lymphoma can be found at NCCN.org/PatientGuidelines and on the NCCN Patient Guides for Cancer app.

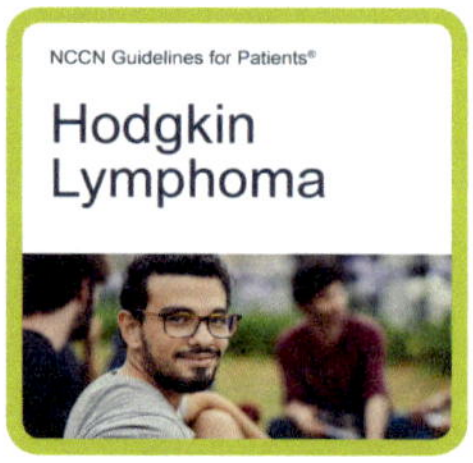

"

It is essential to have a doctor that you trust implicitly, and who knows that you are the ultimate decision-maker in your treatment regimen. If you can't advocate for yourself, ask a family member or friend for help.

– Dixie

Key points

- Tests of biomarkers are needed before starting treatment. New biomarkers may appear during watch and wait or after first-line therapy.
- The preferred first-line therapy is a regimen with a BTK inhibitor or venetoclax. Other options may be chemoimmunotherapy or CD20 antibody treatment.
- The goal of treatment is to achieve a remission and stop CLL from growing.
- Supportive care is an important part of your cancer care. It can help prevent life-threatening infections.
- If first-line therapy doesn't work, you may receive a different type of treatment. For a relapse, your doctor may give the same or a different treatment than was given before.
- CLL can transform into a faster-growing cancer. Clinical trials, chemotherapy, and immunotherapy may be options if this happens.

We want your feedback!

Our goal is to provide helpful and easy-to-understand information on cancer.

Take our survey to let us know what we got right and what we could do better.

NCCN.org/patients/feedback

6
Making treatment decisions

It is important to be comfortable with the cancer treatment you choose. This choice starts with having an open and honest conversation with your care team.

t's your choice

1 shared decision-making, you and your care eam share information, discuss the options, ınd agree on a treatment plan. It starts with an pen and honest conversation between you ınd your team.

'reatment decisions are very personal. What s important to you may not be important to omeone else.

Some things that may play a role in your lecision-making:

- What you want and how that might differ from what others want
- Your religious and spiritual beliefs
- Your feelings about certain treatments like transplants
- Your feelings about side effects
- Cost of treatment, travel to treatment centers, and time away from school or work
- Quality of life and length of life
- How active you are and the activities that are important to you

'hink about what you want from treatment.)iscuss openly the risks and benefits of specific eatments and procedures. Weigh options and hare concerns with your doctor. If you take the time to build a relationship with your team, it will help you feel supported when considering options and making treatment decisions.

Second opinion

It is normal to want to start treatment as soon as possible. While cancer should not be ignored, there is time to have another cancer care provider review your test results and suggest a treatment plan. This is called getting a second opinion, and it's a normal part of cancer care. Even doctors get second opinions!

Things you can do to prepare:

- Check with your insurance company about its rules on second opinions. There may be out-of-pocket costs to see doctors who are not part of your insurance plan.
- Make plans to have copies of all your records sent to the doctor you will see for your second opinion.

Support groups

Many people diagnosed with cancer find support groups to be helpful. Support groups often include people at different stages of treatment. Some people may be newly diagnosed, while others may be finished with treatment. If your hospital or community doesn't have support groups for people with cancer, check out the websites listed in this book.

Questions to ask

Possible questions to ask your cancer care team are listed on the following pages. Feel free to use these or come up with your own. Be clear about your goals for treatment and find out what to expect from treatment.

Questions about cancer testing

1. What tests will I have?
2. Do the tests have any risks?
3. Will my insurance pay for all of the tests you are recommending?
4. Do I need to do anything to prepare for testing?
5. Should I bring someone with me to the appointments?
6. Where do I go for testing, and how long will it take?
7. If any of the tests will hurt, what will you do to make me comfortable?
8. How soon will I know the results and who will explain them to me?
9. How can I get a copy of the pathology report and other test results?
10. Is there an online portal with my test results?

Questions about leukemia

1. What type of leukemia do I have?
2. Is this a fast- or slow-growing leukemia?
3. What is the Rai stage? Does this stage mean the leukemia is advanced?
4. Does the leukemia have any biomarkers? If yes, what do they mean?
5. Do I have to start treatment right away?
6. What can I do to be healthy if I don't need treatment right away?

Questions about treatment options

1. What are my treatment options?
2. Is a clinical trial an option for me?
3. What will happen if I do nothing?
4. Are you suggesting options other than what NCCN recommends? If yes, why?
5. How do my age, sex, overall health, and other factors affect my options?
6. What if I am pregnant, or planning to become pregnant?
7. Does any option offer a cure or long-term cancer control?
8. What are the side effects of the treatments?
9. How do I get a second opinion?
10. How long do I have to decide about treatment, and is there a social worker or someone who can help me decide?

Questions about what to expect

1. Does this hospital or cancer center offer the best treatment for me?
2. Do I have a choice of when to begin treatment?
3. How long will treatment last?
4. Will my insurance cover the treatment you're recommending?
5. Are there any programs to help pay for treatment?
6. What supportive care and services are available to me and my caregivers?
7. Who should I contact with questions or concerns if the office is closed?
8. How will you know if treatment is working?
9. What are the chances of the cancer worsening?
10. What follow-up care is needed after treatment?

Questions about side effects

1. What are the possible complications and side effects of treatment?
2. Does the cancer itself cause any side effects?
3. Which side effects are most common and how long do they usually last?
4. Which side effects are serious or life-threatening?
5. Are there any long-term or permanent side effects?
6. What symptoms should I report right away, and who do I contact?
7. What can I do to prevent or relieve the side effects of treatment?
8. Do any medications worsen side effects?
9. Do any side effects lessen or worsen in severity over time?
10. Will you stop or change treatment if there are serious side effects?

Questions about clinical trials

1. Do you recommend that I consider a clinical trial for treatment?
2. How do I find clinical trials that I can participate in?
3. What are the treatments used in the clinical trial?
4. Has the treatment been used for other types of cancer?
5. What are the risks and benefits of this treatment?
6. What side effects should I expect and how will they be managed?
7. How long will I be in the clinical trial?
8. Will I be able to get other treatment if this doesn't work?
9. How will you know if the treatment is working?
10. Will the clinical trial cost me anything?

Resources

Cancer Hope Network
cancerhopenetwork.org

CLL Society
CLLSociety.org

Lymphoma Research Foundation
lymphoma.org/aboutlymphoma/cll

NCCN Patient and Caregiver Resources
NCCN.org/patientresources

The Leukemia & Lymphoma Society (LLS)
LLS.org/PatientSupport

U.S. National Library of Medicine Clinical Trials Database
clinicaltrials.gov

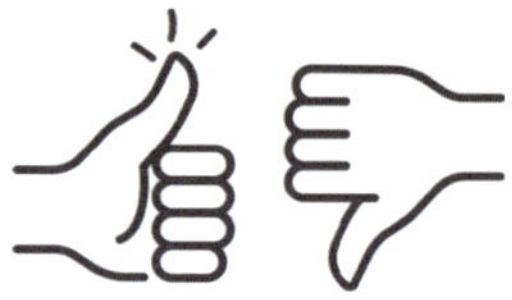

Let us know what you think!

Please take a moment to complete an online survey about the NCCN Guidelines for Patients.

NCCN.org/patients/response

Words to know

ALL
acute lymphoblastic leukemia

allogeneic stem cell transplant
A cancer treatment that replaces abnormal blood stem cells with healthy donor cells. Also called allogeneic hematopoietic cell transplant.

AML
acute myeloid leukemia

anemia
A health condition in which hemoglobin is low.

antibody
A protein in blood that helps fight off infection. Also called an immunoglobulin.

ASO-PCR
allele-specific oligonucleotide polymerase chain reaction

autoimmune hemolytic anemia
An attack on red blood cells by the disease-fighting (immune) system.

B cell
A type of a white blood cell called a lymphocyte. Also called a B lymphocyte.

beta-2 microglobulin
A small protein made by many types of cells.

biopsy
A procedure that removes fluid or tissue samples to be tested for disease.

bone marrow
The sponge-like tissue in the center of most bones.

bone marrow aspiration
A procedure that removes a liquid bone marrow sample to test for a disease.

bone marrow biopsy
A procedure that removes bone and solid bone marrow samples to test for a disease.

B symptoms
A set of symptoms caused by some B-cell cancers.

BCR
B cell receptor

BTK
Bruton's tyrosine kinase

cancer stage
A rating of the outlook of a cancer based on its growth and spread.

chemotherapy
Cancer drugs that stop the cell life cycle so cells don't increase in number.

chromosome
The structures within cells that package DNA and coded instructions for cell behavior (genes).

clinical trial
A type of research that assesses how well health tests or treatments work in people.

CLL
chronic lymphocytic leukemia

CML
chronic myeloid leukemia

omplete blood count (CBC)
lab test that measures the number of red lood cells, white blood cells, and platelets.

omprehensive metabolic panel
ab tests of up to 14 chemicals in your blood. lso called comprehensive chemistry panel.

omputed tomography (CT)
test that uses x-rays from many angles to ake a picture of the insides of the body.

ontrast
dye put into your body to make clearer ictures during imaging tests.

eoxyribonucleic acid (DNA)
chain of chemicals in cells that contains oded instructions for making and controlling ells. Also called the "blueprint of life."

iagnosis
n identification of an illness based on tests.

ifferential
lab test of the number of white blood cells for ach type.

LBCL
iffuse large B-cell lymphoma

chocardiogram
test that uses sound waves to make pictures f the heart.

COG
astern Cooperative Oncology Group

atigue
evere tiredness despite getting enough sleep hat limits one's ability to function.

CR
ludarabine, cyclophosphamide, and rituximab

DA
ood and Drug Administration

fertility counselor
An expert who helps people to have babies.

flow cytometry
A lab test of substances on the surface of cells to identify the type of cells present.

fluorescence in situ hybridization (FISH)
A lab test that uses special dyes to look for abnormal chromosomes and genes.

gene
Coded instructions in cells for making new cells and controlling how cells behave.

GVHD
graft-versus-host disease

HDMP
high-dose methylprednisolone

hemoglobin
A protein with iron in red blood cells.

HLA
human leukocyte antigen

imaging
A test that makes pictures (images) of the insides of the body.

immune system
The body's natural defense against infection and disease.

immunoglobulin
A protein that is made by B cells to help fight off infection. Also called antibody.

immunohistochemistry (IHC)
A lab test that finds specific cancer cell markers involved in abnormal cell growth.

immunomodulator
A cancer drug that modifies some parts of the body's disease-fighting system.

karyotype
A lab test that makes a map of chromosomes to find defects.

lactate dehydrogenase (LDH)
A protein in blood that helps to make energy in cells.

lymph
A clear fluid containing white blood cells.

lymph node
A small, bean-shaped, disease-fighting structure. Also called lymph gland.

lymph vessel
A small tube-shaped structure through which a fluid called lymph travels.

lymphatic system
A network of organs and vessels that collects and transports a fluid called lymph.

lymphocyte
One of three main types of white blood cells that help protect the body from illness.

lymphoma
A cancer of white blood cells called lymphocytes that are within the lymph system.

mantle cell lymphoma
A cancer of B cells that have too many proteins called cyclin D1.

medical history
A report of all your health events and medications.

monoclonal antibody
A type of cancer drug that targets surface proteins on cells.

MRD
minimal residual disease

multigated acquisition (MUGA) scan
A test that uses radiation to make pictures of the heart.

next-generation DNA sequencing (NGS)
A lab test used to detect abnormal changes in DNA.

observation
A period of testing for changes in cancer status while not receiving treatment.

pathologist
A doctor who's an expert in testing cells and tissue to find disease.

performance status
A rating of one's ability to do daily activities.

physical exam
A study of the body by a health expert for signs of disease.

PI3K
phosphoinositide 3-kinase

positron emission tomography (PET)
A test that uses radioactive material to see the shape and function of body parts.

prognosis
The likely course and outcome of a disease based on tests.

pure red cell aplasia
A health condition in which the number of young red blood cells is very low.

purine analog
A drug that prevents the DNA "building blocks" labeled A and G from being used.

Rai staging system
A rating scale of the outlook of chronic lymphocytic leukemia.

eticulocyte
young red blood cell that is formed in bone narrow and is present briefly in blood.

ichter's transformation
change from a slow-growing leukemia into a ast-growing lymphoma. Also called Richter's yndrome.

ide effect
n unhealthy or unpleasant physical or motional response to treatment.

LL
mall lymphocytic lymphoma

pleen
n organ to the left of the stomach that helps rotect the body from disease.

upportive care
lealth care that includes symptom relief but ot cancer treatment. Also called palliative are.

umor lysis syndrome
health condition caused by the rapid death of nany cancer cells.

ric acid
chemical that is made when cells and certain aten food break down.

accine
biological agent that is inserted into the body prevent a disease.

NCCN Contributors

This patient guide is based on the NCCN Clinical Practice Guidelines in Oncology (NCCN Guidelines®) for Chronic Lymphocytic Leukemia, Version 1.2023. It was adapted, reviewed, and published with help from the following people:

Dorothy A. Shead, MS
Senior Director
Patient Information Operations

Laura J. Hanisch, PsyD
Patient Information Program Manager

Susan Kidney
Senior Graphic Design Specialist

The NCCN Clinical Practice Guidelines in Oncology (NCCN Guidelines®) for Chronic Lymphocytic Leukemia, Version 1.2023 were developed by the following NCCN Panel Members:

William G. Wierda, MD, PhD/Chair
The University of Texas
MD Anderson Cancer Center

*Jennifer Brown, MD, PhD/Vice-Chair
Dana-Farber/Brigham and Women's
Cancer Center

Jeremy S. Abramson, MD, MMSc
Massachusetts General Hospital
Cancer Center

Farrukh Awan, MD
UT Southwestern Simmons
Comprehensive Cancer Center

*Syed F. Bilgrami, MD
Yale Cancer Center/Smilow Cancer Hospital

Greg Bociek, MD, MSc
Fred & Pamela Buffett Cancer Center

Danielle Brander, MD
Duke Cancer Institute

*Randall S. Davis, MD
O'Neal Comprehensive
Cancer Center at UAB

Herbert Eradat, MD, MS
UCLA Jonsson
Comprehensive Cancer Center

*Christopher D. Fletcher, MD
University of Wisconsin
Carbone Cancer Center

Sameh Gaballa, MD
Moffitt Cancer Center

Armin Ghobadi, MD
Siteman Cancer Center at Barnes-
Jewish Hospital and Washington
University School of Medicine

Muhammad Saad Hamid, MD
St. Jude Children's Research Hospital/
The University of Tennessee
Health Science Center

Francisco Hernandez-Ilizaliturri, MD
Roswell Park Comprehensive Cancer Center

Brian Hill, MD, PhD
Case Comprehensive Cancer Center/
University Hospitals Seidman Cancer
Center and Cleveland Clinic Taussig
Cancer Institute

Paul Kaesberg, MD
UC Davis Comprehensive Cancer Center

Manali Kamdar, MD
University of Colorado Cancer Center

Lawrence D. Kaplan, MD
UCSF Helen Diller Family
Comprehensive Cancer Center

Nadia Khan, MD
Fox Chase Cancer Center

Thomas J. Kipps, MD, PhD
UC San Diego Moores Cancer Center

Shuo Ma, MD, PhD
Robert H. Lurie Comprehensive Cancer
Center of Northwestern University

Anthony Mato, MD
Memorial Sloan Kettering Cancer Center

Claudio Mosse, MD, PhD
Vanderbilt-Ingram Cancer Center

Stephen Schuster, MD
Abramson Cancer Center
at the University of Pennsylvania

Tanya Siddiqi, MD
City of Hope National Medical Center

Deborah M. Stephens, DO
Huntsman Cancer Institute
at the University of Utah

Chaitra Ujjani, MD
Fred Hutchinson Cancer Research Center

Nina Wagner-Johnston, MD
The Sidney Kimmel Comprehensive
Cancer Center at Johns Hopkins

Jennifer A. Woyach, MD
The Ohio State University Comprehensive
Cancer Center - James Cancer Hospital
and Solove Research Institute

J. Christine Ye, MD, MSc
University of Michigan Rogel Cancer Center

NCCN Staff

Mary Dwyer, MS
Director, Guidelines Operations

Hema Sundar, PhD
Manager, Global Clinical Content

* Reviewed this patient guide. For disclosures, visit NCCN.org/disclosures.

NCCN Cancer Centers

bramson Cancer Center
t the University of Pennsylvania
hiladelphia, Pennsylvania
00.789.7366 • *pennmedicine.org/cancer*

ase Comprehensive Cancer Center/
niversity Hospitals Seidman Cancer
enter and Cleveland Clinic Taussig
ancer Institute
leveland, Ohio
00.641.2422 • UH Seidman Cancer Center
hhospitals.org/services/cancer-services
66.223.8100 • CC Taussig Cancer Institute
y.clevelandclinic.org/departments/cancer
16.844.8797 • Case CCC
ase.edu/cancer

ity of Hope National Medical Center
uarte, California
00.826.4673 • *cityofhope.org*

ana-Farber/Brigham and Women's
ancer Center | Massachusetts
eneral Hospital Cancer Center
oston, Massachusetts
17.732.5500 • *youhaveus.org*
17.726.5130
assgeneral.org/cancer-center

uke Cancer Institute
urham, North Carolina
88.275.3853 • *dukecancerinstitute.org*

ox Chase Cancer Center
hiladelphia, Pennsylvania
88.369.2427 • *foxchase.org*

red & Pamela Buffett Cancer Center
maha, Nebraska
02.559.5600 • *unmc.edu/cancercenter*

red Hutchinson Cancer Center
eattle, Washington
06.667.5000 • *fredhutch.org*

untsman Cancer Institute
t the University of Utah
alt Lake City, Utah
00.824.2073 • *huntsmancancer.org*

diana University
elvin and Bren Simon
omprehensive Cancer Center
dianapolis, Indiana
88.600.4822 • *www.cancer.iu.edu*

Mayo Clinic Cancer Center
Phoenix/Scottsdale, Arizona
Jacksonville, Florida
Rochester, Minnesota
480.301.8000 • Arizona
904.953.0853 • Florida
507.538.3270 • Minnesota
mayoclinic.org/cancercenter

Memorial Sloan Kettering
Cancer Center
New York, New York
800.525.2225 • *mskcc.org*

Moffitt Cancer Center
Tampa, Florida
888.663.3488 • *moffitt.org*

O'Neal Comprehensive
Cancer Center at UAB
Birmingham, Alabama
800.822.0933 • *uab.edu/onealcancercenter*

Robert H. Lurie Comprehensive Cancer
Center of Northwestern University
Chicago, Illinois
866.587.4322 • *cancer.northwestern.edu*

Roswell Park Comprehensive
Cancer Center
Buffalo, New York
877.275.7724 • *roswellpark.org*

Siteman Cancer Center at Barnes-
Jewish Hospital and Washington
University School of Medicine
St. Louis, Missouri
800.600.3606 • *siteman.wustl.edu*

St. Jude Children's
Research Hospital/
The University of Tennessee
Health Science Center
Memphis, Tennessee
866.278.5833 • *stjude.org*
901.448.5500 • *uthsc.edu*

Stanford Cancer Institute
Stanford, California
877.668.7535 • *cancer.stanford.edu*

The Ohio State University
Comprehensive Cancer Center -
James Cancer Hospital and
Solove Research Institute
Columbus, Ohio
800.293.5066 • *cancer.osu.edu*

The Sidney Kimmel Comprehensive
Cancer Center at Johns Hopkins
Baltimore, Maryland
410.955.8964
www.hopkinskimmelcancercenter.org

The University of Texas
MD Anderson Cancer Center
Houston, Texas
844.269.5922 • *mdanderson.org*

UC Davis
Comprehensive Cancer Center
Sacramento, California
916.734.5959 • 800.770.9261
health.ucdavis.edu/cancer

UC San Diego Moores Cancer Center
La Jolla, California
858.822.6100 • *cancer.ucsd.edu*

UCLA Jonsson
Comprehensive Cancer Center
Los Angeles, California
310.825.5268 • *cancer.ucla.edu*

UCSF Helen Diller Family
Comprehensive Cancer Center
San Francisco, California
800.689.8273 • *cancer.ucsf.edu*

University of Colorado Cancer Center
Aurora, Colorado
720.848.0300 • *coloradocancercenter.org*

University of Michigan
Rogel Cancer Center
Ann Arbor, Michigan
800.865.1125 • *rogelcancercenter.org*

University of Wisconsin
Carbone Cancer Center
Madison, Wisconsin
608.265.1700 • *uwhealth.org/cancer*

UT Southwestern Simmons
Comprehensive Cancer Center
Dallas, Texas
214.648.3111 • *utsouthwestern.edu/simmons*

Vanderbilt-Ingram Cancer Center
Nashville, Tennessee
877.936.8422 • *vicc.org*

Yale Cancer Center/
Smilow Cancer Hospital
New Haven, Connecticut
855.4.SMILOW • *yalecancercenter.org*

Index

Made in the USA
Monee, IL
05 November 2026

67379447R00036